NATURAL ACNE SOLUTION

How I Cleared My Acne and Post Acne Scars. Help Teenagers Treat Acne Problem and Cure Grown Ups from Adult Acne and Hormonal Acne

By Ori Laor

Copyright © 2017 by Ori Laor

All rights reserved. No part of this publication may be reproduced, distributed, or transmitted in any form or by any means, including photocopying, recording, or other electronic or mechanical methods, without the prior written permission of the publisher, except in the case of brief quotations embodied in critical reviews and certain other noncommercial uses permitted by copyright law.

ISBN: 978-1981277636

Copyright © 2017

Disclaimer

The methods described within this eBook are the author's personal thoughts. They are not intended to be a definitive set of instructions for this project. You may discover there are other methods and materials to accomplish the same end result.

This book is not intended to be a substitute for the medical advice of a licensed physician. The reader should consult with their doctor in any matters relating to his/her health.

Before beginning any new exercise program, it is recommended that you seek medical advice from your personal physician.

The information contained within this eBook is strictly for educational purposes. If you wish to apply ideas contained in this eBook, you are taking full responsibility for your actions.

The author has made every effort to ensure the accuracy of the information within this book was correct at time of publication. The author does not assume and hereby disclaims any liability to any party for any loss, damage, or disruption caused by errors or omissions, whether such errors or omissions result from accident, negligence, or any other cause.

Thank you very much
Ori Laor

Table of Contents

Personal Introduction 1

    About Me 3

Chapter 1: Pimples Evolution... 5

    Genetic Factor.. 5

    Prevent Pimples 7

    The Reasons 9

    Why Me? 11

Chapter 2: Stress.. 13

    Reduce Inflammation... 13

    Tips to Reduce Stress 14

Chapter 3: Nutrition 17

    The Connection 17

    Foods to Avoid.. 17

    Good Food 21

Chapter 4: Skin Care 25

    Oral Medications 34

    Acne Therapies... 40

    Scars Treatment.. 42

Treating Children 51

Advice for Parents 52

Chapter 5: Break the Cycle 55

Mind Control 55

Adult Acne 56

Makeup Skills 59

Chapter 6: Acne Home Remedies 62

Keep it Natural 62

Conclusion 65

Personal Introduction

Thank you for downloading this fantastic guide - "How to Clear Acne from grown-ups and adults, Hormonal Acne and Post Acne Scars." I cured my Acne myself and learned over the years all it takes to treat Acne efficiently and naturally.

As a child and grown up I suffered from Acute Acne and spent all my time and money looking for cures and answers. This journey made me what I am today a well know Aesthetician Who Helps people and grown-ups take care of their skin problems.

I wrote this book to help people to achieve a clean skin from signs and scars of acne. In this book, I will review all the methods I found capable of treating all kind of Acne at all Ages including Hormonal Acne in mature women.

Acne by the chines starts from an internal heat, so we will try to calm down the heat in our body and mind and find the way to vanish the Acne forever. These pimples appear with beautiful people and very talented ones, and it is connected to passions and heat we produce internally. Acne is a visual skin problem that hearts our self-esteem so by boosting our self-esteem we can fight acne and get our clear skin back.

Acne is an annoying problem to young teenagers and men and women of all age it is a genetic problem but because we live in a world with a lot of pollution and chemicals it is very common to all parts of society.

The key to treat Acne is understanding the cycle of pimples what brings them and what keeps them away for a start your diet your positivity and your skin regime program, you will get all the information in this book.

Acne is connected to food, Stress, Hormone changes, Genetics and your character and social skills, For Example, Feelings can also start the Acne cycle, like feeling miserable and unwanted initiate the chain of our body to make pimples, so we will have a reason to believe that its true. People who treat their skin from a young age tend to be more connected to their body needs, and their skin will tend to get older much slower than others over the years, so there are some comfort in Acne.

In This book, I will take your hand and guide you throw everything you need to do to stop your Acne fast and efficient. I will help you achieve efficiently and naturally the most important steps to make your face clear of pimples and signs of scars and how to always feel and look your best.

For my new Kindle readers, I offer a Free Voucher Gift of 20$. You can find a keyword at the end of this book. Please send it to my mail orilaor@outlook.com, and you will receive a discount for any porches you make for yourself, a member of your family or a friend in LAOR website www.laorcare.com.

About Me

I have a passion for Beauty, Skincare, Anti-aging and well-being methods. In my extensive exploration around the world, I gathered sacred pieces of information that helped me and then other people from all walks of life to look and feel younger. I hold a BA in Art and diplomas for Makeup Artist, Para Medical Aesthetician, Aromatherapy, Naturopathy, and Nutrition consultant. I am a well-known name in T.V scene and in the cosmetic industry, including treating many celebrities. When I was 30 years old, I quit working for others and founded LAOR, a House of natural Beauty and Professional Skin Care and treatments for the face, Body, and Mind.

Since an early age, I suffered from my skin and was carried away with Skincare research, science and well-being. I worked in beauty and style departments in New York and Tel Aviv, based on my experience I invented a revolutionary practice for treating the skin from within – **The Layer system**, Complied with a line of professional cosmetic products and treatments for the face to treat any skin problem.

Ientered the natural cosmetics world with a unique world-view and with one simple, honest purpose: to create a different kind of cosmetic that is Natural and effective. My desire is that each product would provide each with the essence of beauty, based on effective ingredients.

Now, for the past Two Decades, I am designing the products that Men and women across the world love, helping them to look and feel younger with all the secrets of skin care. When I am not working, I love to design and create, read, write and paint. My quest is to bring more beauty to the world and raise self-awareness.

Let's Get Started!

Chapter 1

Pimples Evolution

Genetic Factor

Most cases of Acne in young and teenagers show an immediate connection to one of the parent's or grandparents. For Example: in most cases, if the father or mother had Acne the child has more statistic possibility to have Acne too.

The acne starts from an inflammation in the skin, inflammation can start from bad food and also from bad thoughts and sadness it is important to keep our self-happy most of the time to reduce inflammation, sport and yoga are an excellent way to clean our thoughts and the physical body. Remember Positivity can overcome genetic Acne. So it is crucial to balance the skin physically and mentally everyone must strive to find is own way to self-calmness. I will talk about that much later in the book.

The origin of pimples/acne is still unknown. Nobody exactly knows why the pores in some people start to produce excessive oil and inflammation or in short pimples.

Nevertheless, it is now known that a change in nutrition and some professional cosmetic treatments can help.

Acne is a skin disease, which is created by the clogged pores on the skin. It is a major problem for millions of teenagers, both male and female. The cure is not one thing but a holistic approach to life with changes to a more healthy lifestyle.

Though pimples are just a small bump on the skin, the effects could be traumatic on some, as we can lose self-esteem when we have major pimples problem. It is advised to get it treated with the help of a dermatologist who would recommend proper treatments, which would help heal and prevent acne, and a nutritionist to select the right food to lower inflammation as I will describe later.

Proper care like cleaning the face and use professional skin care like Azelaic Acid and Retinol creams in the morning and before bedtime are recommended. Shaving properly with natural soaps and not the regular SLS soaps that close the pores, avoiding the sun to minimize scaring and choosing the right natural and professional cosmetics would help a lot to get this perfect skin.

Acne is a condition which ninety percent of the population goes through in their teenage years. For some, this condition continues until their middle age too. Never plucks the acne as it could leave a mark on your face. The best way to counter this condition is by being health conscious and maintain a skin care regime with proper products for Acne, which I will examine in this book. I will show you all the new and effective ingredients you need to fight your Acne fast.

Prevent Pimples

How to prevent pimples are usually the first major problem and concern of adolescents. During the period of maturity, pimples are commonly seen on several exposed parts of the human body like the face, shoulder, neck and even on the back. Most often than not, pimples are considered a nightmare, and it even affects the sociability of an individual especially the teenagers.

Pimples are unusual inflammations or even swelling of the epidermal layers. They are usually varied in sizes as there are big and smaller pimples. Pimples have proven by dermatological experts that they emerged on the skin due to irritation to some environmental elements like dust. Dust can easily cause pimples to appear because it clogs the pores.When dust enters the holes on the outermost layering of the skin called epidermis, it will block the holes and eventually irritate the interior and more delicate parts that cause it to swell and inflame.

Another Known cause of pimples is through extracting the pimples, not by a professional Aesthetician. Trying to play with the pimples not professionally want to eliminate them and probably will make the situation even worse due to excessive production of the sebaceous gland after treating the pimples not the right way.

The sebaceous gland functions as a lubricator of the skin as it produces and eventually secretes oils to a different part of the body and in some cases cause Acne. Some parts of the human body often experience excessive and over production of oils especially in the chest region, some parts of the face specifically between the nasal region and all over the facial part of the human body. The produced oil of the sebaceous gland will pass through the follicular region or tiny pathways up to the outermost part of the skin or epidermis. Originally, the oil cycle secreted by the sebaceous gland stored up in the most endothermic part of the skin. Germs and dirt can lead to irritation of the endodermic part of the skin, and this will eventually cause pimples to appear. So cleaning and exfoliating the skin is crucial.

The skin of young people who are likely to grow pimples is mainly caused by their hormones. The hormone element produced by their body makes the sebaceous glands produce excessive sebum which leads to dead skin cells clogging up and increasing the probability of pore blockage. The best way to balance hormones is a good natural diet, especially dairy free and NO junk food.

The Reasons

In some people's genes it is programmed to produce more sebum such a skin type is referred to as oily. In some cases, there is a frequent shedding of dead skin that intervenes with hair follicles and causes a blockage. Hence three major factors lead to the formation of acne.

- Sebum overproduction

- Irregular accumulation of dead skin interfering with hair follicles

- Accumulation of bacteria

Acne breakouts are tentative when your hair follicles get clogged. The two-agents responsible for causing this blockade are the dead skin cells, and oily secretion called sebum. Since your hair follicles end in a sebaceous gland, thesecretion helps to keep the hair lubricated. When it is released, sebum travels along the hair shaft up to the surface of your skin. It happens normally, but when there is the excess release of sebum or the dead skin cells pile-up, this build up can lead to a plug that facilitates an environment for bacterial growth like infection is most likely to occur. In severe cases of acne, infection pustules are formed. Initially, the blockade creates a slight bulge, and you have a white head. In case, this plug is exposed to the surface, and it gets darkened.

Some form of pimples are the red colored spots that are developed over some time when the hair follicles are infected and inflamed. When these inflammation and blockages are not cured, it can go deep and create lumps under the skin. It might be surprising to note that your sweat gland pores also opening over your skin are not involved in acne.

When, the sebaceous glands, located at the base of hair follicles, become overactive, pimples breakout. Moreover, those sensitive and vulnerable parts of the body, such as the face, back, chest and shoulders, have the likelihood of growing pimples. The most common pimple is "pimple vulgaris" which happens mainly at puberty. Youths need to learn how to take precautions to prevent dirt or excessive oil from building so as not to attract bacteria growth on their skin; otherwise pores become infected, red spots are visible and can lead to skin scars.

Many causes produce pimples, but we need to learn how pimples grow then we need to take the proper methods to prevent acne from growing and developing.

Why Me?

Of course, people vary in different ways. Often, a pimple free face is a subject of envious to many especially for girls regardless of age. It is nothing but a common concern for youths in their early maturity and development in dealing with pimples. However, who usually get easily affected with pimples? Is it a particular case for a specific age group?

Well, this is always wrong because pimples can be into everybody. Having pimples is associated with different human bodily functions. Example, people who are prone to pimples are experiencing the so called hormonal imbalance. People can get over the years food allergies to any thing from peaches to milk and gluten and develop skin disorders. Obisity sometimes leads to pimples. In addition, women of any age can lose the hormone balance for many reasons and start to develop acne.

Adolescents are the most prone to pimples. As they mature, their human systems, as well as their hormones, begin to develop and even functions abnormally. Teens are known to be aggressive in all things and activities that cause some of the hormones to undergo into additional features. When Bacterium Propionibacterium enters the scene, it will further develop intosevere case called acne.

If you have inherited acne from your family, the onset begins in your early teens. Just like the color of your eyes is your destiny, acne is inevitable if it's in your genes. However, wait, don't get disheartened yet because there is another side of the equation. The good news is this part of the equation is somewhat under your control.

Chapter 2

Stress

Reduce Inflammation

Stress is the main cause for Acne in any age it increases inflammation and disturbs the hormone balance which disturbs the balance in the body. All kind of meditation can help calm down the inflammation. Inflammation is made by internal heat, so its nice to lower the flames by having a mantra or listening to soft and relaxing music.

In this fast-paced society, it is hard to avoid stress in our daily lives. But letting this stress accumulate in your body can have disastrous effects. In studies that have been conducted, researcher's have found that stress can raise the production of cytokines, which cause inflammation to occur. An increase in the body's inflammatory response can lead to a higher risk of conditions that are related to inflammation.

Emotional turmoil and stress can cause the body to produce an overabundant number of hormones. Male hormones especially have a great impact on the sebaceous gland. If the gland becomes overactive, the body then producestoo much sebum. Sebum can clog the hair follicles on the face and body and create acne as a result.

In addition to aggravating current acne breakouts, stress can also cause an overall decline in the appearance of your skin. Besides affecting sebum production, an unhealthy amount of stress may cause the adrenal glands to produce cortisol. The cortisol then is released into the sebaceous gland and provides a greater amount of oil in the skin.

Even if you're currently taking a prescription or over the counter treatment for acne, reducing your stress level can help to improve your overall skin condition. The following tips are helpful for reducing stress to combat acne. By following some of these suggestions, not only will your acne likely improve but you can also achieve better overall health and wellness.

Tips to Reduce Stress

One of the steps to take to stop inflammation so you can get rid of your acne breakouts is to take the supplement of Omega 3 from vegetarian source or fish. Fish oil has has been called by scientists as nature's most potent anti-inflammatory.

Adding a powerful Omega 3fish oil supplement or Omega 3 from a vegetarian source like chia seeds is one of the best ideas you can take to reduce the amount of inflammation and acne you have. While you can increase the oily fish that you eat to help add more fish oil, usually it is best to go with fish oil supplements so that you get the amount that your body needs to eliminate inflammation and reduce acne adequately.

Exercise -Is perhaps one of the best-known methods for reducing stress. Finding an exercise or activity that you like to will help keep you faithful to maintaining a routine. In a matter of minutes, you can alleviate excess tension and anxiety.

Watch your diet - Try to eat as many healthy and natural foods as possible. A food containing the proper amount of fruits and vegetables can have the most positive impact on your health. By changing your eating habits, you can improve your acne dramatically, and I will discuss that later in the book.

Sunshine - Getting the sun can have a positive effect on your body. Sunshine exposure is responsible for stimulating the production of Vitamin D which promotes healthy skin. A short walk several times a week is all that is needed.

Too much caffeine - Can often result in a high level of stress. By reducing your intake of sodas, coffee, tea, and other stimulants, you can both calm your body and prevent other common adverse side effects such as headaches or an increase in heart rate.

Of course, stress cannot always be avoided certain life events carry with them a certain amount of uncertainty, anxiety and hard work, with common causes of stress including things like a moving house, relationship changes, bereavement and the loss of a job.

Acne Products - It is most unlikely that you will be able to avoid stress responses when major events occur in your life, however being aware that these can affect your acne can help you ensure you take extra care of your skin at these times and have your preferred professional acne treatment on hand.

<u>Chapter 3</u>

Nutrition

The Connection

The Food is The Major Couse for Acne. Some people can eat anything and have no pimples some other people who do suffer from pimples has to be more restricted with the food. If you want to stop the Acne, you have to take brave actions in your life. Don't eat Gluten it clogs the digestive system so more toxins go out from the skin and not from the digestive system. No dairy products they stimulate the production of sebum in the skin they also increase inflammation in the body and feed the bacteria that start the pimples. Reduce Sugar intake from any source for balancing the hormone system. It is recommended to take Omega 3 capsules and Magnesium and periodically Zinc.

Foods to Avoid

What you eat can affect your skin in both big and small ways. The wrong diet can be a contributing factor that gets in the way of your clear skin. We hear a lot about the problems of the western diet of fast foods and processed foods in the media, but here are some eating habits that we should specifically avoid.

High-glycemic foods- Are high up on the list, especially for men. These are foods that are highly processed, and among them, pieces of bread are one of the most common elements in the western diet, although certainly not the only. High-glycemic foods include processed grains, refined sugars, and many dairy products.

A good way to judge the potential threat of a portion of food is to consult a Glycemic Index (GI), which is readily available online. This way you can find out if any of these foods are unwittingly playing a major part in your diet.

But what is it about high-glycemic foods that are so bad for your skin? Glycemic foods earn their name because they affect your body's blood-sugar levels. These foods bring about an increase in insulin levels and also the growth factor IGF-1. This, in turn, leads to a dramatic increase in the production of the male growth hormone testosterone. With overproduction of testosterone come excess levels of sebum (skin oil), and excess sebum is the cause of most acne.

Between bread and cereals, processed grains, in particular, are a significant element of the western diet. Many carbohydrates that are not even considered junk food can still have adverse effects on your skin. It has been backed up by several studies, and also telling is the fact that many cultures and regions that have a low intake of processed grains have dramatically lower rates of acne. Does this mean you should avoid all bread. Certainly not, but substituting rice or the occasional whole grain food is a good idea. Moreover, this type of evidence brings us back to the fact that conquering acne is ultimately about managing your body's output and metabolism of skin oil. Sebum is the real problem behind most acne, not bacteria or any dirt or grime on the surface of your skin. Acne starts from the inside, and you need a skin care regimen that stops it from the inside if you're going to find lasting results. Much of this evidence consistently strengthens the central tenant of vitamin B5 acne theory that by reducing skin oil (by increasing sebum metabolism or decreasing sebum production) you can ultimately put a real stop to acne.

If your acne is proving stubborn despite all the treatments you've tried, try taking a hard look at your diet. Use a Glycemic Index to identify what specific foods diet may be causing you trouble by raising your insulin levels. Put reasonable limits on your intake of these foods, and don't just cut out carbohydrates from your diet altogether, but find healthy alternatives to processed grains.

Cheese - Dairy products are believed to be the worst foods if you are trying to avoid acne. Cheese is enriched with a high level of fat and as you have learned, too much fat can cause acne.

Milk - Almost all the time, it is extracted from cows that are pregnant. Unfortunately, their milk contains hormones. Skin glands of people have enzyme containing organs which convert the certain hormones to Dihydrotestosterone. It boosts oil production and leads to acne.

Sugar and refined carbohydrates - These often cause blood sugar issues. They enter the bloodstream rapidly, and the blood sugar levels are beingspiked up. Too much fat aggravates the problem. It will eventually lead to acne and other deficiencies.

Gluten - Any food with Gluten and remember not to eat Gluten free products they are much worse for you as they contain Corn and Sugars. If you take for example Pizza, a mix of Gluten and dairy, its greasy and highfat. It is often agreed to be responsible for acne outbreaks. Anthropologist's have come up with the term sympathetic magic. It dictates a belief of "like causes like." The best explanation for this is, if you eat pizza, you will look like a pizza.

Any food with caffeine - Caffeine increases production of hormones and leads to acne or worse, more acne. It contains a high level of toxins which manifests as acne once it escapes through the skin.

Good Food

What we eat affects every organ in our body. Simply put, the food we consume causes chemical changes that affect our body's condition. Different kinds of food can have different effects on our skin too. In fact, some types of food have been found to make skin healthier and even help with acne. Here is a list of the top five foods for more radiant, blemish-free skin.

Green Leafy Vegetables - If we just listened to mom when we were kids, eating more lettuce, broccoli and cabbage would have made our skin look flawless and beautiful. It is because green leafy vegetables are packed with antioxidants that boost skin health, prevent wrinkles and dark spots, and help pimples heal faster. If you are out for the best green veg for your skin, pick spinach. Not only is it packedwith antioxidants, but it's also rich in other skin-boosting vitamins and minerals like vitamin A, zinc, magnesium, and vitamin E.

Berries - The berry family of fruits is another skin secret. Ancient Greeks are said to regularly use a skin clearing mask of crushed berries with goat milk. And it's no wonder why berries are very rich in skin-boosting antioxidants, vitamins, and minerals. Blueberries, in particular, are a good source of fiber, vitamin A, vitamins C, riboflavin, and vitamin E. These nutrients are not just good for the body but excellent for the skin too. Other skin-friendly members of the berry family include raspberries, blackberries, and strawberries.

Grapefruit - Like most other citrus fruits, grapefruits are rich in the antioxidant vitamin C., Unlike oranges and lemons. However, grapefruits are also packed with vitamins A and B -vitamins known to boost skin health and improve the appearance of both wrinkles and pimples. That is why the lowly grapefruit stands way above its citrusy brothers. And a good reason why you should incorporate it into your daily diet too.

Carrots - Bugs bunny may not have known it, but munching on carrots can be one of the surest ways to clearer, smoother skin. This vegetable takes its name from beta carotene, a pigment that is a precursor to vitamin A. Vitamin A is used in many skin and acne products to reduce pimple redness and inflammation, manage hyper active oil glands, and even reduce fine lines and wrinkles. Other foods rich in beta carotene include squash, pumpkin, and mangoes.

Turmeric - possesses anti-oxidant and anti-inflammatory properties, which are both beneficial in treating acne.Turmeric for treating skin disorders has been used for centuries in Eastern and Asian countries.Turmeric made into a paste and applied to acne-prone areas can destroy the P.acnes bacteria that cause inflammation and remove excess oil from the skin. You can download a good Turmeric recipe in my free kindle book enclosed.

Water - Okay, so technically water is not food. But it is the best thing you can consume for clearer, healthier skin. Why? Water flushes out all the toxins and impurities from the skin. Skin cells also need water so that they can heal faster, be suppler, and be better protected from infection, damage, and irritation. It also helps that water has zero calories too and is more beneficial to your body than sugar-laden sodas or alcoholic drinks.

Chapter 4

Skin Care

Treatment Products

In the decades that the prevalence of acne has exponentially surged, so have the number of treatments available. The various products available at the economic level is astounding in itself. You have exfoliating scrubs, alcohol pads, home dermabrasion kits, foaming washes, Professional products, and Pharm Products, the list goes on and on. At the professional level, you have laser treatments and prescription medications. Acne treatment work by balancing the skin and by reducing oil production, speeding up skin cell turnover, fighting bacterial infection or reducing inflammation which helps prevent scarring.

When you wish to buy a product for your Acne make sure it is Natural with no chemicals and make sure it includes one or more of the ingredients below. At LAOR www.laorcare.com we provide natural and professional products that are well tested on thousands of people and not on animals and can give you all the answers you need to treat your skin.

Topical Medications - These products work best if you buy them from professional aesthetics centers and not from a pharma store. You may not see the benefit of this treatment for few weeks. And you may notice skin irritation at first, such as redness, dryness, and peel.

Aha Acid Face wash and Exfoliators - Alpha Hydroxy Acids (AHA) which are primarily extracted out of fruits can act as excellent solvents for dirt and oil. They can efficiently cleanse the outer layers of the cell. They can remove acne marks like scars and blackheads.

AHA, face washes can be used twice a day both during morning and evening. For pore clearing, AHA (Alpha Hydroxy Acid) is fantastic. It sloughs off the dead skin cells that would otherwise clog up the pores. The ones the skin doctors administer unclog the pores

We need exfoliators because our Skin is always turning over, generating new cells at the lower level (the dermis) and sending them up to replace dead skin cells with the upper layer (epidermis). As we get older, the cell turnover process slows down. Cells begins to gather unevenly on the skin's surface which can lead to dry patches and tired looking skin. Through exfoliating your skin, we can help to remove dead skin cells, revealing the fresher, younger cells below and restoring skin's natural clarity and brightness.

Some people prefer to exfoliate their face in the mornings because they claim that makeup sits better. Others would rather prefer to exfoliate their face & body in the evening to remove dead skin cells and dirt. So really, just pick a suitable time for you as long as you exfoliate.

Glycolic and Lactic Acids - Keep Your Skin Breathe, Glycolic acid has been proven to be effective in removing acne scars, evening out color tones of the skin and provide an overall smoother complexion.

Glycolic acid is a fruit derivative coming from the family of Alpha-Hydroxy acids. What makes this component compelling is the fact that it's the smallest of the AHA relatives.

It can penetrate deep into the pores of the top dermis layer to bring dead skin cells to the surface. It is also known for promoting collagen and elastin production. Think of it as a highly skilled gardener whose purpose is to identify and eliminate weeds and insects that can destroy its beauty, while at the same time nurturing the rest of the flowers living together from beneath the soil.

According to reports made to the FDA alpha-hydroxy acids in large quantities have been known to cause itching, peeling, severe irritation, dermatitis or rash. Less than 14% has been established to be a safe practice. Anything exceeding that amount will require your doctor's supervision.

Some treatments such as Glycolic Acid peels that could contain up to 70% concentration causes damage to the top layer of the skin, forcing it to heal and regenerating while eliminating acne scars.

AHA has been known to increase the sensitivity of the skin to ultraviolet light. It also has has been found that this sensitivity is not permanent, the skin returns to its original condition sometime after its prolonged exposure. It is always important to use a moisturizer containing sun screen to protect yourself during the glycolic acid treatment

Many dermatologist's advise doing them once a week for approximately 6 or 8 procedures after which letting your skin rest. Start with a 10% peel and do it for two weeks, after that you can increase it to 20% and then 35% and then 50 and 70% for maximum advantages.

When applying glycolic on your face, make sure to stay away from hypersensitive regions like your nostrils or under-eye area. Let the acid stay on your face for a minute or so depending on the intensity of the peel. After putting it on you might feel a stinging sensation but that's normal.

After you wash it off, you might notice that your skin is red, but the redness will become less within one day. The use of makeup and sunscreen is necessary if you wish to go out-of-doors or to any social functions right after a glycolic peel since it helps to cover any remaining reddishness.

Salicylic acid - Is another ingredient that works by unclogging the pores. This is a much harsh ingredient a part of the old world of treating Acne.

Retinoids and Azelaic Acid - Thisbest combination of ingredients comes as creams, gels, and lotions. Retinoid is derived from vitamin A. You apply this medication in the evening, beginning with three times a week, then daily as your skin becomes used to it. It works better if it is combined with Azelaic Acid in the product or a separate product, the Azelaic acid works on the inflammation.

Retinoid Acid - Vitamin A is used as an ingredient in certain medicines. Vitamin A is found very useful to treat non-inflammatory types of acne on face. It can open clogged pores. Retinoids reduces the excess production of skin oil causing Skin to become dry. Due to this fact Retinoids are also prescribed for oral use to treat severe cases of acne because it over all reduces the excess production of oil. Retinoids also have certain harmful side effects. Retinoic acid can help your skin in several ways: Improve tone by distributing melanin, Reduce wrinkles by boosting collagen production, Decrease collagen breakdown, Fight sun damage, Fight acne, Speed cell turnover rate, Shrink pores.

Azelaic Acid - Azelaic acid is a natural chemical that's produced by the action of a particular yeast. It is a naturally occurring acid that may be found in grains like wheat. This chemical has three main and very distinct properties that have elevated its role in acne treatment: The ability to fight off anaerobic bacteria (P. acnes) that cause the pustules and lesions on the face, back, neck and chest. The ability to reducing inflammation (though its relative strength is small compared to specially designed anti-inflammatory products). It also can decrease the number of comedones in affected areas.

Tea tree oil - kills the bacteria and is very antiseptic. For boils, applying a drop of tea tree oil on each boil every 2-hours may be enough to kill the bacteria and bring down the boil.

Clay Masks to Purify the Skin - One product thatalways gives best results is the clay mask. This affordable treatment, which, is often advertised in magazines and on television, is designed to help, reduce oil levels. It can eventually lead to drastic reduction in the number of new breakouts.

Acne occurs when one of the pores on our skin becomes clogged with debris. These contaminants are primarily composed of dead skin, which in an acnefree individual are disposed of regularly by the skin. The obstruction keeps oil from flowing to the surface of the skin, allowing it to collect inside instead. Inside the pore, you also have Acnes bacteria which use oil (or sebum) as food. With such an abundance of food sources, they were to multiply rapidly and eventually produce an acne lesion. Clay masks can help eliminate the oil which is involved in the acne equation, leaving you with clear skin. When the bacteria have nothing to feed off of, they cannot duplicate. You can also reap some other aesthetic benefits from using a clay mask, including no longer having to put up with an oily complexion.

You will often discover different information when it comes to how and when to use a clay mask. Since it can be drying, it's often a good idea to limit usage to a maximum of twice or three times a week. You need to follow the instructions provided for your particular product carefully. They should specify how long to leave the mask on before washing it off. Skin irritation may arise for failing to adhere to instructions.

You should use clay mask at night since your skin's absorption ability is improved at that moment of time. Apply the clay evenly over your face after you wash your face properly. Relax and wait for 10-15 minutes or as instructed by the instruction. Wash your face, and your skin will feel very smooth. There are other more creative ways to mix clay mask with other remedies. For example, you can mix clay mask with lemon juice, honey, apple cider vinegar and so on. To treat your acne, using clay mask and lemon juice is the better combination.

Antibiotics–All Antibiotics come with a prescription formula that you can get from a doctor, thesework by killing excess skin bacteria and reducing redness. For the first few months of treatment, you may use both a retinoid and an antibiotic, with the medicine applied in the morning and the retinoid in the evening.

Antibiotics for acne work in four main ways. First, they fight acne causing bacteria. It helps to reduce the number of acne causing bacteria on the skin and therefore to help reduce the breakouts. Also, the antibiotics contribute to preventing the recurrence of the breakouts by protecting the skin from the acne causing bacteria. Secondly, they actively unclog skin pores by removing any particles and dirt which might cause the acne.

Topical antibiotics usually do this. They contain exfoliant ingredients which help to unclog skin pores and remove any dead skin cells. Thirdly, they reduce histamine in the blood. Histamine is produced by the white blood cells as animmune response leading to inflammation. Finally, the antibiotics help to maintain a hormonal balance within the body. Hormone imbalance has been linked to excessive sebum secretion in the oil glands which contributes to the development of acne breakouts.

Topical Antibiotics For Acne - These antibiotics are applied directly to the affected area. They come in the form of lotions, gels, pads, ointments, and creams. Application of the antibiotics usually comes after thoroughly cleaning the skin. Anyone with acne breakouts can use antibiotics for acne as a treatment method. However, given the possible side effects and some conditions such as pregnancy, skin disease, and other health related conditions, it is best to consult a dermatologist before taking any of these antibiotics.

Oral Medications

Oral Antibiotics - For moderate to severe acne, you may need oral antibiotics to reduce bacteria and fight inflammation. You will likely use topical medications and oral antibiotics together. Antibiotics may cause side effects, such as an upset stomach and dizziness. These drugs also increase your skin's sun sensitivity. Antibiotic treatment is not magic, and sometimes the body gets amuned to it very quickly and the treatment stop to work, so never replace natural foods, professional face products and healthy lifestyle with any drug.

Antibiotics work by selectively killing the bacteria. They do not cause damage to the cells of the body. By killing the bacteria, antibiotics reduce the infection and inflammation. Oral antibiotics are the fastest way to treat such diseases. The common antibiotics used for this are- Erythromycin, Tetracycline, Minocycline, Doxycycline, Clindamycin, and others.

Erythromycin - It is a broad-spectrum antibiotic. It is available in capsule, tablet, long-acting capsule, long-acting tablet forms. It is commonly prescribed to be taken two to three times a day for seven or more days. The strength and the dosage duration depend upon the severity of the infection. It can be used in pregnancy. It not only reduces disease, but also reduces inflammation. It istaken along with or after food. Erythromycin may cause diarrhea, upset stomach, vomiting, etc. If such side effects persist, you need to consult with your doctor.

Tetracycline - It is another antibiotic that is very commonly used to treat acne. Tetracycline is commonly available as a capsule. The strength and the dosage duration depend upon the severity of the infection. Tetracycline cannot be taken during pregnancy. It should be taken on an empty stomach and should not be made with any milk products. It can cause side effects such as- sore mouth, skin redness, diarrhea, upset stomach, etc.

Minocycline - Minocycline belongs to the class of medications known as tetracycline antibiotics. Minocycline is commonly available as a capsule or a tablet. The strength and the dosage duration depend upon the severity of the infection. Tetracycline cannot be taken during pregnancy. It should be taken on an empty stomach and should not be taken with any milk products. It can cause side effects such as- sore mouth, skin redness, diarrhea, ringing in ears, etc.

Doxycycline - Doxycycline also belongs to the class of medications known as tetracycline antibiotics. It is available as capsule or tablets. If you feel nausea with Doxycycline, take it with food or milk. The strength and the dosage duration depend upon the severity of the infection. Doxycycline may cause dry mouth, diarrhea, and sunburns.

Clindamycin - Clindamycin is used as an antibiotic for acne, but because it may cause colitis, it is commonly employed in the topical form. If your doctor has prescribed Clindamycin oral, discuss the side effects in detail.

Oral Isotretinoin (Accutane) -This medicine is reserved for people with the most severe acne. I don't recommend to take it but you should now all the information and decide for yourself. Isotretinoin is an Oral Retinoid powerful drug for people whose acne does not respond to other treatments. Oral isotretinoin is very effective. But because of its potential side effects, doctors need to monitor anyone they treat with this drug carefully.

When all else have failed, go back to check your diet habits. But if you want to move on to the most popular oral remedy for acne: isotretinoin you should know its dangers. In the United Kingdom and the United States, the original brand name is still the most widely known: Accutane. Yes, the same Accutane that was reported to have caused depression to some people.

Before you quake with fear, let's sift through the product. Then, you can proceed to your doctor and discuss what you think of the product before you get a prescription for it.

There are several key problems when a person engages in the long-term use of isotretinoin: *Increased incidence of suicide and depression in users, High probability of non-hereditary congenital disabilities in the unborn.It can lead to dryness in the skin for life, it* *can arouse other skin problems like Seborrheic dermatitis and psoriasis.*Milder side effects like dry lips are persistent and irritating.

Now that you are aware of what could happen to you let's discuss what isotretinoin is capable of carrying out as an anti-acne agent.

Unlike other modes of treatment, isotretinoin has been known to make acne in a conventional treatment lasting fifteen weeks or twenty weeks.

Because of its popularity as an anti-acne drug, this retinoid is closely monitored in the United States. Dermatologists are of the opinion that if patients follow medical precautions correctly, there shouldn't be any problems. The point? Don't take more than what's prescribed! Remember, when you ingest isotretinoin, it becomes a teratogen. Teratogenic substances cause malformations in unborn children. Never take undue risks when pregnant. Consult with your doctor first.

When taken orally for a prescribed period, isotretinoin does the following: First, it affects the sebum production. Sebum production is slowed down, cutting off the food supply of the harmful anaerobic organisms hiding in the blocked pores of the skin. It makes oral isotretinoin a drying agent. Next, isotretinoin regulates and normalizes the keratinization of the skin. When a person has acne, the skin sheds its outer layer far too oftenWhen this happens, the small pores in the skin become blocked. By fixing the keratinization of the skin, you avoid comedones formation. Comedones are the white heads and black heads you see on your nose.

You may consider using this product for the following reasons: If you have severe nodular acne, If you have inflammatory acne, If you have severe acne that keeps recurring. If you are experiencing mental stress because of your acne, in whatever form it has takenIt is important the person taking isotretinoin and for their family members to be educated regarding the potential for mood swings and depression during isotretinoin therapy. In most cases, psychosocial events associated with severe acne most often improve once the acne starts to clear.

However, in some people with acne who, have depression or a tendency toward depression, their psychologic outlook does not improve with acne treatment. It may be due to several different reasons. However, oral isotretinoin should be discontinued in these cases, and treatment should be instituted for the depression as needed.

Some physicians believe that oral isotretinoin does produce, very occasionally bet unpredictably, significant psychiatric side effect. It is essential to discuss these issues with your doctor and also to let your doctor know whether you have been treated in the past for depression or suicide attempts or whether you have a family history of depression.

Tip: It may take a few weeks for acne treatments to reach their fullest potential. Some acne treatments may take six-to eight weeks before their results are seen. In some cases, treatment may even cause acne to become worse before helping to reduce it. Patients should speak with their doctor or skin care professional for more specifics on treatment duration and effectiveness so that they may gain a thorough understanding of their options.

Acne Therapies

These therapies may be suggested in select cases, either alone or in combination with medications.

Light Therapy - A variety of light-based therapies has been tried with success. Further study is needed to determine the ideal method, light source, and dose. Light therapy targets the bacteria that cause acne inflammation. Some types of light therapy are done in the dermatologist Clinique. Blue-light therapy can be done at home with a hand-held device.

Recently Light therapy for acne has shown to be a promising break through. It works by utilizing a blue or a red-light wave. The FDA has approved this process for mild to moderate acne. Light therapy for acne, involves exposing the skin to the light for about 20 to 30 minutes, And uses a blue ray to destroy the bacteria Propionibacterium.

The red light used in light therapy for acne helps to reduce the swelling and inflammation caused by the white blood cells. Some patients do have some mild pain after using light therapy.

You can get Light therapy for acne and treatments are often offered through a dermatologist center. It usually takes the form of monthly treatments as acne is an ongoing problem for many. There are now hand-held devices available that can be purchased for the home.

It is recommended that it is discussed with a doctor about these to see which would work the best for the type and severity of acne you are suffering from

Beauty Treatment - Extraction of whiteheads and blackheads. Your dermatologist uses specialized products to gently remove whiteheads and blackheads (comedones) that haven't cleared up with topical medications. It is important to have a regular treatment to keep skin clean. The face treatment helps balance the skin and treat the inflammation.

Steroid Injection - Steroidal injections may be the last option if your cysts do not respond to anything else. They primarily involve a doctor placing a liquid steroid into the affected area, which can reduce inflammation and infection.

It is vital for both the patient and the dermatologist to review the procedures as to the treatment of acne scars. Choosing a skin rejuvenation process is based partly on the result that the patient wants to accomplish.

Scars Treatment

When your acne goes away, it leaves horrid marks on your skin. People will say to you that these are temporary and will fade away with time but believe me they are there to stay. If you do not take any treatment plan, then youcannot get rid of them. Derma Rollers or Pen is the easiest and very effective treatment plan against your acne marks or scars whatever you call them.

Derma Roller - The best way to treat Acne scars at home or professionally is using at least once a week a roller or derma pen at least 0.5 mm and even after a while to use 0.7 mm Roller. It is best to use Retinol and Azelaic acid after the treatment to get the skin renew itself from within and eliminate scaring and pigmentation.

Derma Roller or Pen with its effective way of handling your skin removes the scars from your face and neck. Some people also get acne on their hands and arms, which leave some marks there too which makes them wear full sleeve shirts. But with the use of Derma Rollers or Derma Pen, you can wear anything you want.

You can complete the treatment completely by yourself, from the comfort of your home. It's a one-time fee to purchase a product like this, and you won't have to break your budget. A derma roller is completely risk-free, meaning you have nothing to worry.

So, if you're looking for the best in acne scar treatment and removal, then a derma roller is the answer to your prayers. It's a highly effective form of micro needling which will allow your body to heal itself naturally.

It starts to work immediately, and you will begin to see results in no time at all. Put your hard-earned money into something else, and save your time and energy for other chores. You can fix your acne scars without a high cost or any hassle, and the results will speak for themselves.

Soft Tissue Fillers - Injecting soft tissue fillers, such as Hyaluronic Acid or fat, under the skin and into indented scars can fill out or stretch the skin. It makes the scars less noticeable. Results are temporary, so you would need to repeat the injections periodically. Side effects include temporary swelling, redness and bruising.

Self-fat Injections - This method of acne scar healing revolves around the removal of other tissues from another part of the body and using them to fill the gap left by acne scars. Self-fat injection act like Soft tissue fillers, such as Restylane, Perlane, and Juvederm, are non-animal-based hyaluronic acid (HA) used to correct and restore volume loss (deflation) and to hydrate the skin.

Skin Peels - This procedure uses repeated applications of the professional solution, such as salicylic acid and AHA Acids. It is most effective when combined with other acne treatments, except oral retinoids. Deep peels aren't recommended for people taking oral retinoids because together these treatments can significantly irritate the skin. Deep peels may cause temporary, severe redness, scaling and blistering, and long-term discoloration of the skin.

Deep peels are the most intensive type of chemical peels available. Because active chemicals are used, deep peels are only available from qualified dermatologist's or plastic surgeons. Although the results are beneficial, the discomfort levels which are experienced during this type of peel can also be high and will leave the skin looking "sunburnt" during the recovery process.

Deep peels are only recommended for those who already have deep age lines and wrinkles, or who have pronounced scarring. Deep peels can be very effective in treating these problems. Most people who choose deep peels will do so on the professional advice of a trained skincare expert.

A deep skin peel is applied to the skin for 20-30 minutes. They can be made up of many ingredients or concentration that has several different ingredients in its formula. Gold is one favorite ingredient due to its antioxidant properties and perceived value. If you visit a high-end spa around the world, chances are you will see a gold skin care mask or facial treatment.

Alpha hydroxyl acid Peel (AHA) is the mildest and widely used of all chemical peels since it is mostly made from natural components. It works by exfoliating the skin, loosening, and eventually removing the layer of dead cells on the skin surface. It usually takes longer to see results given that it is a mild chemical peel.

Beta hydroxyl acid Peel (BHA) has become more popular and seen to be used increasingly for chemical peel treatments instead of AHA peels. It has shown to work deeper into the skin, control oil and remove dead skin cells better than AHA peels. Salicylic acid is an excellent example of BHA.

Retinoic peel is a procedure which must be performed by a qualified professional in the clinic. It is a deep peel and usually done along with a Jessner peel. It is very effective in eliminating scars, wrinkles, and uneven spots.

Jessner peel is a solution of lactic acid and 14% salicylic acid in resorcinol with an ethyl alcohol base. "Skin over peel" is a very rare possibility when using a Jessner peel because the ingredients used are in tiny percentages.

Phenol Peel is considered the strongest type of peeling, and it is not common these days due to its side effect and the sensitivity it leaves the skin for months after the treatment. It is also the type that delivers the most satisfying results. It is readily the peel recommended to treat various scars, deep wrinkles, and aged skin. Although it produces results, it will take time for the skin to recoveras it works deeper into the skin surface. It also increases the risk of hyperpigmentation.

Trichloroacetic Peel is the type that stands between the AHA and the Phenol peels. It produces results for almost all skin types. It delivers moderate skin peeling, improvement of uneven skin tone, and fine wrinkles.

Although chemical peel is a safe procedure, sure people experience permanent or temporary color change of their skin. Many people also get scars on some areas of their face after undergoing this procedure. Chemical peeling is very beneficial for those individuals who suffer from various skin problems, but before undergoing this procedure, it is highly essential for you to consult a skin specialist.

Dermabrasion - This procedure is usually reserved for more severe scarring. It involves scrubbing the surface layer of skin with a rotating brush. It helps blend acne scars into the surrounding skin. Dermabrasion merely is put; a procedure which utilizes manual abrasion of the skin to remove acne scarring. The damaged outer layers of skin are gradually removed. The skin then slowly regenerates over time. Full dermabrasion will be performed by a surgeon or doctor.

The procedure does not take very long, perhaps an hour or so, but it can be excruciating. The doctor uses a small, fast rotating implement to reduce the visibility of the scars. The end of this tool has a metal wheel which has a rough surface. Before the procedure is carried out an anesthetic must be given. It can be general or local. Afterward, the patient's face will be red and raw.

The good news is that for many acne scarring sufferers a full dermabrasion treatment such as this not required. There are now available on the market many home products, often coming under the heading of microdermabrasion, which can be only applied by the user in the comfort of their surroundings.

Micro dermabrasion islight dermabrasion. It has been referred to as the lunchtime facial. As the name indicates micro dermabrasion limits itself to removing only the top skin layer. It then reveals the fresh, undamaged skin below.

The ease of the treatments means that the face does not become sore in the same way as with a full dermabrasion procedure. Micro dermabrasion could be called a type of specialist exfoliation. It should leave the skin feeling fresh and damp. Lines and of course can be scarring are gradually reduced with treatment.

Laser Resurfacing - It is a skin resurfacing procedure that uses a laser to improve the appearance of your skin. The impact of lasers on the medical and dermatological field has been tremendous, and through laser resurfacing, patient's have new, and efficient options. Treating acne and acne scars have become a primary concern of many young men and women. Adult acne and acne scars in adult's leave many patients searching for options. Thanks to a growing field, patient's have at least one more efficient option for treatment.

The use of lasers in the medical and dermatological field has grown tremendously in the past 20 years. The effect that this technology has had on the medical field has been massive. Lasers are used in many facets of the field from cosmetic procedures such as acne treatment to its application in the main surgeries.

Using lasers, doctors can burn the top layer of skin and promote the growth of new skin and collagen. This process, known as laser resurfacing, has been effective in reducing acne scarring in many patients. In some cases, laser resurfacing is combined with other treatments such as chemical peels, dermabrasion, and collagen injections, although in many cases laser resurfacing has replaced these other options.

Available lasers and specifics about their effectiveness, patients should speak with a skin care professional. Redness and tenderness may be possible side effects in the days following treatment.

Most often than not, the result of laser surfacing can be seen on the face within a few weeks of the treatment. During this time, you will notice the formation of a new skin on your face.

The rejuvenated and fresh skin that you get on your face is a result of the formation of this new skin.

Treating Children

Because the food is poisoned, and children are eating fries and dairy products, children often from 9- 10 years old especially girls start to have new acne. It is better not to start with medication but to start changing the food and clean their plates from junk food and especially dairy products.

Acne cure is essential for those affected by acne. We all know that acne is a major problem with teens, although it can affect anyone. However, the teenagers are the hardest hit with this issue. Teens tend to go through substantial psychological effects with this problem. It is during adolescence that one gives most priority to looks and if at during this time you are affected by acne, it becomes a matter of concern.

Many teens that develop acne get conscious about this issue and avoid social interactions or any other kind of activity. If this happens, they tend to become introverted and may affect the development of their personality significantly. Many reasons could lead to acne like incorrect diet, infection, unhygienic conditions, etc.

Acne outburst increases with junk food, oily foods, sweets, and drinks. To combat acne, the first thing is to look at diet consumption and hygienic conditions. For proper acne cure, you must visit a dermatologist to understand the cause. A medical professional will analyze your lifestyle and suggest treatments accordingly. There are many topical treatments also available which are quite capable. It ensures that physically acne gets treated.

Advice for Parents

One of the beautiful things that parents could do is have a chat with their teenage children on this issue. They should be a part through the treatment and try to get the best support possible for the problem to get cured. It will not only boost the self-confidence in your teenage child but will also restore faith between you and the child. Your teenage child needs to understand the temporary nature of acne and how with time it will get cured.

One crucial point that must be shared with the teenage child coping with acne is that no one is concerned about this problem and people do not even notice it. So, the child getting conscious at social gatherings will restore his confidence. In most cases, this problem is temporary, affects almost all of us and vanishes with proper care and treatment.

You as a parent can even go on to explaining how acne occurs, the medical explanation. When this kind of discussion takes place, the teenage child doesnot feel ignorant and will feel better. The best help that a child gets to overcome the Psychological problem is from the parents. No one better can deal with this than you as a parent. It will go a long way with the child in the development of his personality.

Few other important tips must be shared with the teenagers suffering from acne. Such as knowledge about the fact that squeezing the pimples or scrubbing them will only worsen the problem and may leave permanent marks as well. There are different treatments available to cure acne ranging from medical care to diet change. In some severe cases, even drug therapy is administered.

Acne cure can be done with topical treatments as well which are available in the form of creams, lotions, gels available which are quite useful in treating acne. In the case of acne seems to be quite harsh and there is no impact of the topical treatments or any other self-treatment taken, in such cases, a doctor should be consulted immediately.

Finally, one of the most important things you can do to help with your child's acne problems is to be there for him, especiallywith preparing and checking the food he eats. There's a good chance that he will be upset about the difficult problem of acne outbreaks, and he may be looking for some comfort and assurance that things will be okay. It is your job as Parent to help him feel better.

Chapter 5

Break the Cycle

Mind Control

Boys and girls who have Acne must learn to control and have balance in their life, balance reflects on the skin, and when you are out of balance, the skin is out of balance. When one's find inner quit, everything will work correctly in the body. Nice to do Meditation or Yoga or any sports, when you are happy you will forget about the pimples, always look on the bright side of life and free yourself from the vicious cycle of pimples.

It's a never-ending cycle. Sounds terrible but that's just how pimples work. It has been scientifically proven that the mind affects the skin. Worrying and stressing about anything greatly increases the chances of acne to form.

What you need to do right now is take control of your mind. That may sound kind of weird, but it is a definite must. If you find that you worry over every little thing that goes on in your life, you will notice that your acne may never go away.

If you're saying you used to never worry about anything, but now all you do is stress out about your acne, then you know what you need to do. You need to stop stressing out about your acne.

No one will notice your Acne it if you choose to ignore it. Of course, you should still treat it in your spare time but don't let it bog you down. The first step in this battle against acne starts with the mind.

Adult Acne

To understand how to fight adult acne effectively, start by understanding what can cause acne formation. Every one of us adults would want to think we'll never experience those embarrassing pimples ever again. If you are reading this book, you are living proof pimples, and zits don't stop with adolescence.

Recurring adult acne can be just as hard to cope with emotionally as it was when you were younger. Most adult acne sufferers want effective treatments, yet get frustrated when the so called "best acne treatments" don't deliver. There are unknown reasons that your treatment of acne does not leave you acne free. Once you understand the underlying cause of pimples and blackheads, you will see your acne fighting program become more efficient.

When those zits crop up on your face, again and again, they get in the way of life. In addition, it seems like acne appears at the most inconvenient time like the week before your wedding or just before an important presentation. Left uncontrolled, acne is the source of a great deal of emotional trauma. Unless it's handled, it leads to acne induced stress which can keep you away from being in public and even push you toward depression.

Dirty Skin - The fundamental reason acne breaks out is dirty skin. Most of us attack acne at the skin level hoping to improve skin pores clogged with dead skin and excess sebum before acne-causing bacteria can climb into the clogged pores and start an infection. The body's defense system kicks in. The result is unsightly, embarrassing blackheads and whiteheads. The first thought formost of us to apply a topical product like benzoyl peroxide or whatever heavy duty over the counter acne solution we have in the medicine cabinet.

Toxins - that accumulate inside our body also lead to acne formation. Consider these toxins as "dirt" inside the body.

Acne causing toxins stem from food allergies, hormone imbalances, and stress. Daily stress has been shown to increase both the flow from the adrenals and cortisol, the stress hormone shown to increase sebum production.

Most doctors will tell you that food does not directly cause acne. While that may be true, many adults have discovered that certain foods do trigger acne flare ups. Plus, hormonal changes happen as we age. Pregnancy adds to the toxin load, too, because of the enormous shift in hormones during that time. Whenever the body generates toxins, it wants to eliminate them. It's understandable the body's normal cleansing process pushes those toxins toward the skin cells since it's an important part of the excretory system.

For adult acne treatments to be effective, you must reduce the impact of hormone upsets and stress. Watch the foods you eat especially dairy products and in severe cases eliminate gluten from your diet. Write down any foods you believe may lead to outbreaks. Watch for a pattern. If you find one, simply quit eating that food. To reduce stress in your daily life and along with it the hormones that breed acne, the tried and true methods are best: get plenty of rest (8 hours, preferably), take up calming exercise like Yoga or TaiChi and train yourself to mentally detach from the crazy events that make up your life

Makeup Skills

Try to work on your character is the first thing if you are shy try to be out if you are a loud person try to work on you're quitness. Take good care of your face with professional products and don't neglect it will not be better if you don't take the matters into your hand be assertive even when you treat your pimples.

Don't be shy to use makeup to cover the pimples this is why makeup was invented.Acne is, of course, a very disturbing and upsetting condition, but makeup can help you conceal the scars and pimples that are caused by this naturally occurring skin blemish. Makeup is a favorite choice of many people to hide their acne. One of the most important things to consider when choosing makeup to cover acne is that it is appropriate for the condition.

Acne can be made worse by makeup that contains mineral oil, The key to success with this is to choose mineral oil-free makeup. Read the labels to make sure it is mineral oil-free.

Most of your good, brand name products will be oil-free. Using oil-free makeup and cleansing products will ensure that you are not going to aggravate the acne.If you are not sure which is the best to choose, then it is recommended to get some advice from your dermatologist or skin care specialist rather than just guessing. If you have a lot of acne scarring, then there are some special camouflage make-upsavailable nowadays. It can be perfect for concealing scarring and is also made for those with problem skin.

One of the main things to remember when you are using makeup for acne is to make sure that your skin is immaculate and that you use a variety of cleansers that are safe for skin with acne. You should also make sure that when you take off the makeup, you are very careful to make sure that you have taken all of it off. It is essential to make sure that the skin is clear of all makeup so that the pores are clear and do not get clogged up.

One of the most useful types of makeup, when you have acne, is concealer. It is very good for covering up blemishes and also works well on scarring. You need to take care when applying this as it is the basis of your makeup and is a vital ingredient in allowing you to camouflage the acne well. Don't use too thick a layer but just make sure that it is even so that it can work well. You also need to apply a foundation to give your skin a natural appearance to cover the fact that you have been using the concealer to cover your acne and not make it so obvious.

Acne and makeup are very well suited to each other despite what some people think, you just to have to make sure that you look after the skin by keeping it clean and ensuring that you get it all off afterward. It can make the skin seem to be a lot clearer, and this can give the sufferer a lot more confidence, but you need to make sure that buy a makeup that is suited to the condition. If you buy the right makeup and apply it well, then it can make a real difference.

Chapter 6

Acne Home Remedies

Keep it Natural

Because acne is such a common skin problem, there have been many home remedies popping up all over the Internet.

Most people love home remedies for acne because the methods used are often straightforward and cheap. Most of these methods are all natural and can easily be found in either your home or local grocery store. You can download my Natural Beauty Recipies Book and make your own effective products to treat your skin.

Eat healthier - There have been some studies that claim that rich foods can be one of the main causes of acne. So, what you have been eating can be contributing to your acne problem. You should eat healthier non-greasy foods such as fresh fruits and raw vegetables.

Stay clean, stay pure - Always keep your face and your body clean. Get rid of any fragrant soaps that you have, and replace it with an unscented one. As scented soaps often contain chemicals that can irritate skin. Don't use any exfoliators as these are meant to get rid of dry skin, not pimples. Many of these will do more to aggravate your skin than to help it.

All-natural products - One of the great things about using home remedies for acne is that you can use natural products to cure acne.

Clay Mask - A clay facial mask does wonders for any skin. In the case of an acne, regular use of clay masks reduce infection, swelling, and help close the pores while leaving you with glowing skin, you can find an example how to prepare a clay mask in my free Natural recipes book.

Grape Seed Oil - Using pure Grape Seed oil can be a tremendous moisturizer for your skin. It can also be used to heal open wounds that your acne has caused. Using Oil with Oily skin helps balance the production of the sebaceous glands.

Tea tree oil -This oil has a vast amount of medicinal benefits. Just to name a few, it is an antifungal, antiseptic, and antibacterial oil that can be used, quite effectively, against bacteria associated with your acne.

However, this oil can be quite harsh, and it is recommended to dilute a tiny bit with water before applying with a clean cotton ball.

Because of the simplicity and low cost, we can ensure long-term acne treatment which might not be the case if we would pay for existing treatment products and spend a lot of money before we achieve the desired results. By making remedies at home, we can choose the proper solution for our skin condition and continue the treatments until we get rid of acne.

There is also the possibility of complementary treatment where we use several homemade remedies and combine them wisely in our treatment plan to prevent the causes and consequences of our skin problem.

As we have seen, there are many advantages of using home remedies and one should consider which type of treatment is the most suitable for his skin condition. If the traditional solutions do not help you to get rid of acne, then you should try to make your remedy and explore the possibilities of treating acne at home.

Conclusion

Bringing the balance to our lives will restore balance in the face, working on our self-esteem will help us overcome Acne. The food is a crucial element in healing the Acne mainly milk products, Gluten, and Simple Sugars. Keep eating junk food won't help for anything.

Take good care of the face with quality products and treat the scars with a Roller. Acne that comes from genetics can be beaten with good mind healthy foods and by taking good care of our faces with efficient products.

It is essential to repeat here that before you launch into any of these top acne treatments, consult a physician or a skin specialist. It will ensure that you choose the right treatment depending on the type of acne you are suffering from, the type of skin you have and the severity of the acne.

Treating Acne With Laor Products Gives Fast Results And Smooth Facial Skin.

At LAOR, we recommend a combination of active products with professional treatments In Laor center. The professional treatment takes care with the source of the problem and it is supportive with the home care products. The Products are all natural, effective and operate in three easy steps to cure the infection in the subcutaneous glands that is typical to acne. Taking self-Care with the products is easy and does not require a long time, also it have no side effects and the improvement of skin appearance is visible immediately.

Step 1: Cleaning – Is the basis for the prevention of pimples. Keeping the skin smooth require thorough cleansing of the skin. The cleansing step disinfects and removes the dead cells that accumulate every day and block the pores. Accumulation of dead cells in the skin produces oil in the pores and is expressed in pimples. It is recommended to clean the skin with soap 1A and exfoliating product number 8. It is best to complete the cleanup with face disinfectants toner containing alcohol and herbs – product number 4. The clay mask No. 11 is good to use daily to absorb the excess oil from the skin and reducing open pores.

Step 2: Balance – Parra Medical ingredients help to control inflammation and balances the action of the sebaceous glands in the face. Professional Treatment reduces inflammation and addresses the source of the Pimples, contributes to a clear healthy skin. This step supports the deep relaxation of the skin and reduces the production of oil and skin pimples. It is recommended to use daily a balance cream for acne, product No -20 and combine weekly with the use of glycolic solution product No 19P Phase 1 with azelaic acid and the cream from Phase 2 product number 20, to suppress the infection. Propolis extract product No 17 contributes to healing pimples and calming the skin. When the skin feels dry and itchy moisturizer can be integrated like product number 51.

Step 3: Rehabilitation – to maintain the results of home and professional treatments it essential to take care every day from the sun and environmental pollution. Protection from the sun with sunscreen, product number 72, is a critical step to avoid the appearance of spots and pimples and stop the processes of skin darkening and scaring. For topical treatment of pimples nightly, it is advised to use propolis extract with green clay product number 65.

Remember, acne is a preventable, controllable and treatable skin condition as long as you commit to proper care and continuous self-improvement. Instead of getting stressed by the situation, take the initiative and improve your health, your diet, your lifestyle and your self-esteem.

In conclusion, just remember that combination skin acne treatments are the best options if you have combination skin. Products that are designed either for oily or dry skin generally will not produce the most hoped-for results. Yes, treating combination skin acne is probably twice as hard, but with perseverance, implementing a regular skin care routine, using appropriate products, a person can eventually get rid of acne.

Thank you very much for reading the book. If you loved the book, I would appreciate it if you can write a review of the book for me. If you have any question about the book feel free to contact me at orilaor@outlook.com.

For 20$ Coupon for www.laorcare.com were you can find all the professional products to clear your Acne and scars, send the word: YOUCANDOIT to my mail.

With sincere love Ori Laor

www.ingramcontent.com/pod-product-compliance
Lightning Source LLC
Chambersburg PA
CBHW060759260726
48660CB00002B/701